FERTILITY DIET COOKBOOK PLAN FOR WOMEN

Overcoming common obstacles with Nutrition

CAMILA.C.HIL

Book title [FERTILITY DIET COOKBOOK PLAN FOR WOMEN]

TABLE OF CONTENT

Introduction

Introduction

Explanation of the importance of nutrition for fertility

As a woman who has struggled with fertility issues for years, I was desperate for a solution. I tried different medical treatments, therapy sessions, and even spiritual practices. However, I didn't know that my diet could have a significant impact on my fertility.

That's when I discovered the Fertility Diet Cookbook plan for women. This cookbook is based on research conducted by Harvard Medical School and follows the guidelines of the Nurses' Health Study. The plan focuses on certain foods that are known to boost fertility and recommends avoiding others that may negatively affect it.

I was skeptical at first, but after reading through the book and trying out some of the recipes, I noticed a change in my body. I had more energy, my menstrual cycle became more regular, and I even lost a few extra pounds.

The Fertility Diet Cookbook plan is not just about losing weight or limiting certain foods. It encourages a healthy, balanced diet that includes fruits, vegetables, whole grains, and lean proteins, which all have specific nutrients that support fertility.

The recipes in the cookbook are easy to follow and include ingredients that are affordable and accessible. Some of my favorites include avocado and egg toast for breakfast, Mediterranean chicken and vegetable skewers for lunch, and roasted salmon with quinoa and asparagus for dinner.

Overall, I highly recommend the Fertility Diet Cookbook plan for women who are struggling to conceive. Not only does it provide nourishing meals, but it also educates on why certain foods are beneficial and how they can impact fertility. Nutrition plays a crucial role in fertility, as it directly affects the overall reproductive health in both men and women. Proper nutrition ensures that the body is receiving the necessary vitamins and nutrients needed for the growth and development of healthy eggs and sperm.

In women, a healthy diet can improve the quality and regularity of menstrual cycles, increase the production of cervical mucus, and support the overall health of the ovaries and reproductive system. On the other hand, deficiencies in certain vitamins and minerals such as folate, iron, and vitamin D can negatively impact fertility in women by increasing the risk of ovulatory disorders, pregnancy complications, and infertility.

Similarly, in men, adequate nutrition affects sperm production and quality. A diet rich in antioxidants, protein, and folate can increase sperm count, motility and morphology, while deficiencies in these nutrients can lead to infertility.

Moreover, maintaining a healthy weight through proper nutrition is crucial for fertility, as obesity and undernutrition can cause hormonal imbalances, which can negatively affect fertility.

Overall, proper nutrition is paramount for fertility as it can help optimize the chances of conception and improve the chances of having a healthy pregnancy and baby

.

Overview of the book's goals and content

The Fertility Diet Cookbook Plan for Women" is a book written by a renowned reproductive endocrinologist, and nutritionist . The book provides a comprehensive guide on how to use nutrition to boost fertility. The main goal of the book is to help women achieve a healthy weight, improve their hormonal balance, and optimize their chances for conception.

The book starts by explaining the importance of the right diet during a woman's reproductive years. It then provides a detailed plan that is tailored to different stages of fertility, from preconception to pregnancy, giving tips on foods that aid in reproductive health and avoid those that may hinder the process.

In addition, the cookbook provides over 100 nutrient-rich recipes that are delicious and easy to prepare. The recipes are categorized according to meal times and offer diverse options for breakfast, lunch, dinner, and snacks.

Overall, "The Fertility Diet Cookbook Plan for Women" is an excellent resource for women who are looking to optimize their fertility through a healthy diet. It provides scientifically backed information and practical tools to help women navigate the often-complicated world of fertility nutrition.

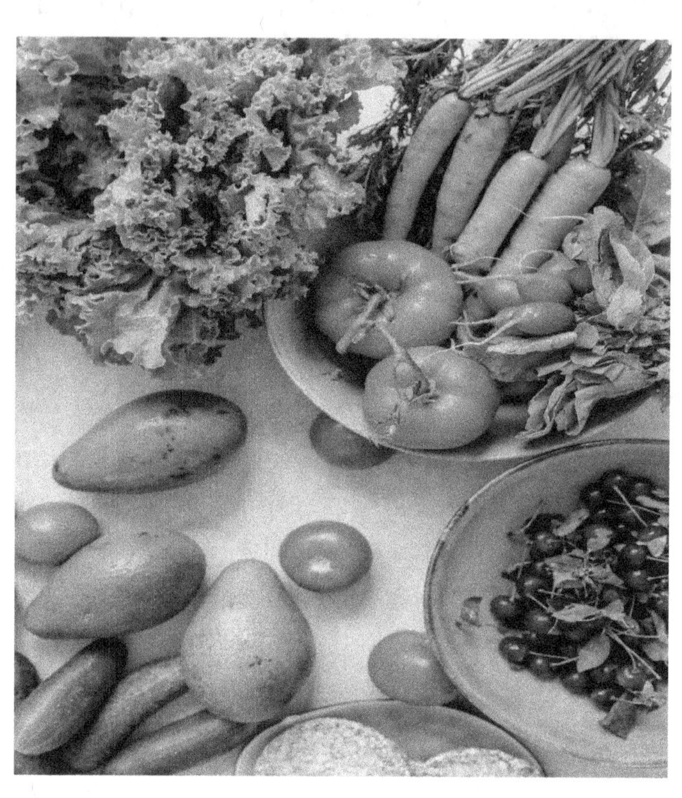

Chapter 1

: **Fertility and Nutrition**

Nutrition plays a crucial role in the fertility and reproductive health of both men and women. In order for the body to function properly, it requires the proper balance of nutrients, vitamins, and minerals. Research has shown that a healthy diet can improve fertility outcomes, while a poor diet can negatively impact fertility.

For women, consuming a diet rich in fruits, vegetables, whole grains, and lean proteins, and low in saturated fats and refined sugars, can improve fertility outcomes. In addition, certain nutrients such as folic acid, iron, and omega-3 fatty acids have been linked to increased fertility and a reduced risk of infertility.

For men, a healthy diet that includes fruits, vegetables, whole grains, lean protein, and healthy fats can improve sperm quality and quantity. Certain nutrients such as zinc, vitamin E, and selenium have been linked to improved sperm health.

However, it is important to note that nutrition is just one factor that contributes to fertility and reproductive health. Other factors such as age, medical history, and lifestyle habits such as smoking and excessive alcohol consumption also play a role. However, here are some general tips that can contribute to optimal fertility and nutrition for women:

1. To maintain a healthy diet, it is important to consume a diverse range of nutritious foods such as fruits, vegetables, whole grains, lean protein, and healthy fats. It is advisable to minimize the intake of processed and high-fat foods.

2. Maintain a healthy weight: Being either overweight or underweight can negatively impact your fertility. Maintaining a healthy

weight can be achieved by combining a well-balanced diet with regular exercise.

3. Get enough essential vitamins and minerals: Nutrients like folic acid, iron, and calcium are important for reproductive health. Make sure to eat foods rich in these nutrients or consider taking a supplement.

4. Stay hydrated: Drinking enough water is important for overall health, including reproductive health.

5. Limit caffeine and alcohol: Too much caffeine and alcohol can interfere with ovulation and overall fertility.

6. Avoid smoking: Smoking can decrease fertility and increase the risk of complications during pregnancy.

7. Manage stress: Stress can affect your menstrual cycle and fertility. It is essential to adopt healthy coping mechanisms to manage stress, such as meditation, yoga or seeking counsel from a therapist.

How nutrition affects fertility

Nutrition can affect fertility in women in several ways. A poor diet and nutritional deficiencies can lead to hormonal imbalances, irregular periods, and ovulation problems that can make it more difficult to get pregnant. Here are some specific ways how nutrition affects fertility in women:

1. Folic Acid: Folic acid is essential for women who are trying to conceive as it helps to prevent birth defects in babies. A deficiency in folic acid can lead to problems such as neural tube defects and miscarriage.

2. Iron: Iron is important for the production of red blood cells and helps women maintain healthy ovulation cycles. Low levels of iron can lead to anemia, which can negatively impact fertility.

3. Vitamin D: Vitamin D helps to regulate hormone levels and aids in implantation of the fertilized egg. Women with inadequate

levels of Vitamin D are more likely to experience infertility.

4. Antioxidants: Antioxidants such as Vitamin C and E can help to protect the ovarian follicles from damage and improve egg quality, thereby increasing fertility.

5. Omega-3 Fatty Acids: Omega-3 fatty acids have an anti-inflammatory effect on the body and can help to improve menstrual irregularities and ovulation, thereby increasing fertility.

Overall, a balanced and nutritious diet, rich in whole foods such as fruits, vegetables, legumes, nuts, and seeds can help to improve fertility in women.

Overview of the best types of foods for fertility

1. Whole grains: Whole grains help regulate insulin and blood sugar levels, which can prevent ovulatory infertility. Whole grains

such as brown rice, quinoa, and whole wheat bread are excellent examples.

2. Leafy greens: Leafy greens like spinach, kale, and broccoli are high in folate and other important vitamins and minerals that support fertility. Fetal growth and development significantly rely on the adequate supply of folate.

3. Fatty fish: Fatty fish like salmon and sardines are high in omega-3 fatty acids, which can boost fertility by reducing inflammation and improving ovarian function.

4. Legumes: Legumes like lentils, chickpeas, and beans are high in protein and fiber, which can help regulate ovulation and improve overall fertility.

5. Berries: Berries like blueberries, raspberries, and strawberries are high in antioxidants, which can protect eggs and sperm from damage.

6. Nuts and seeds: Nuts and seeds like almonds, walnuts, and chia seeds are high

in healthy fats and other nutrients that support fertility.

7. Lean protein: Lean protein sources like chicken, turkey, and tofu are important for overall health and fertility.

It is important to remember that a healthy and balanced diet is key for fertility, and individual needs may vary based on age, weight, and underlying health conditions. For tailored advice, it is recommended to seek guidance from a registered dietitian or healthcare provider.

Nutrients essential for fertility and reproductive health

1. Folic Acid: A B vitamin that can decrease the risk of birth defects in the fetus and also promote fertility in women.

2. Iron: Helps to maintain healthy levels of hemoglobin, which transports oxygen around the body and plays a role in ovulation and fertility.

3. Calcium: Important for maintaining strong bones and may also help regulate menstrual cycles.

4. Vitamin D: Helps the body absorb calcium, maintain bone health, and may have a role in ovulation and fertility.

5. Omega-3 Fatty Acids: Found in fatty fish, flaxseeds, and chia seeds, they have been associated with increased fertility.

6. Zinc: Important for the development and function of healthy eggs and may also help regulate menstrual cycles.

7. Vitamin C: An antioxidant that helps improve overall reproductive health.

8. Vitamin E: Helps improve reproductive health by reducing oxidative stress in the body.

It's important to note that a balanced and varied diet, along with maintaining a healthy weight and lifestyle, is crucial for optimal fertility and reproductive health. It's recommended to consult with a healthcare professional and a registered dietitian for individualized advice.

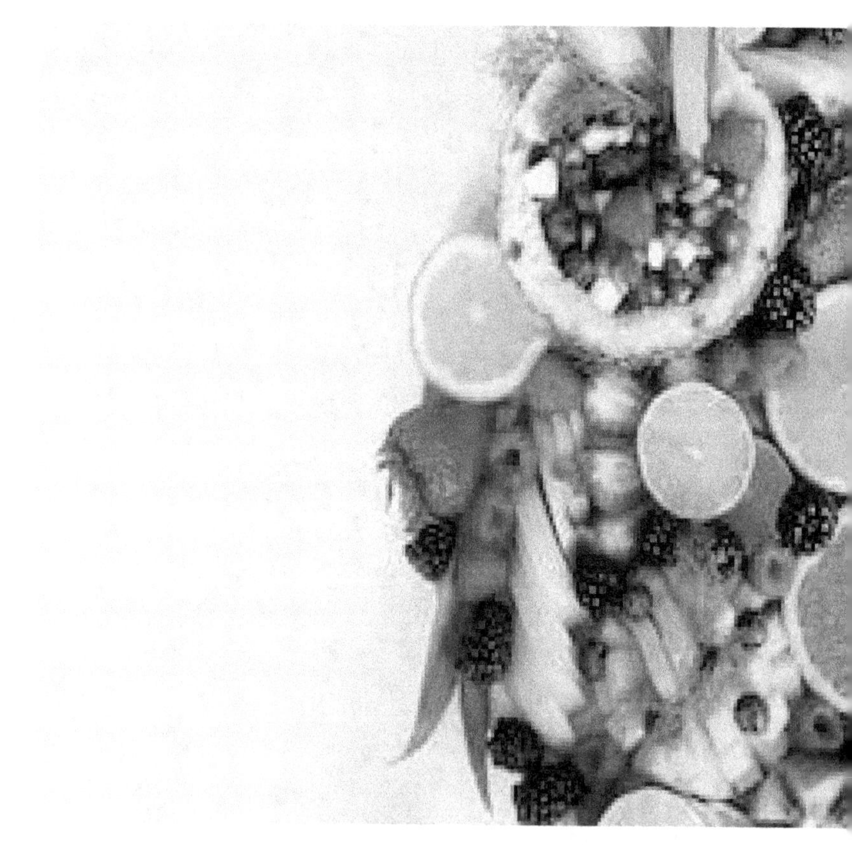

Chapter 2

Fertility Diet Plan

1. Whole grains: These are high in fiber and provide energy and nutrients. Oats, brown rice, and quinoa are some instances of this.
2. Fruits and vegetables: These are rich in antioxidants and vitamins that can help improve fertility. Be sure to incorporate an ample amount of cruciferous vegetables such as broccoli and cauliflower, leafy greens, citrus fruits, and berries into your diet.

3. Lean protein: Women trying to conceive should consume lean protein sources like chicken, fish, and tofu as they provide essential amino acids and are low in saturated fat.

4. Full-fat dairy: Dairy products such as full-fat milk, yogurt, and cheese contain high levels of calcium, protein, and vitamins that can help improve fertility.

5. Nuts and Seeds: Rich in Omega-3 fatty acids, protein and healthy fats, nuts and seeds boost fertility. Some instances of this are chia seeds, flaxseeds, almonds, and walnuts.

6. Healthy fats: Include monounsaturated and polyunsaturated fats such as olive oil, avocado, and fatty fish, as they provide essential vitamins and minerals.

It is advisable to avoid processed foods, refined sugars, and excess caffeine and alcohol in order to improve fertility. It's best to consult a healthcare provider or a registered dietitian to create a personalized fertility diet plan.

Detailed description of the fertility diet plan, including daily meal plans

The fertility diet is a specially designed dietary plan that is meant to improve your overall reproductive health and increase your chances of conceiving a healthy baby.

It includes a variety of foods that are rich in vitamins, minerals, antioxidants, and other essential nutrients that can help to balance your hormones, improve your ovulation, and reduce your inflammation levels.

Here is a detailed description of the fertility diet plan, including daily meal plans:

Breakfast:

Option 1: Smoothie - Blend together 1 cup of almond milk, 1 banana, 1 scoop of protein powder, 1 tbsp of almond butter, and some spinach.
Option 2: Greek yogurt with fruit - 1 cup of low-fat plain Greek yogurt with strawberries, blueberries, and a handful of nuts.
Option 3: Oatmeal - Cook 1/2 cup of rolled oats with almond milk topped with sliced bananas, a spoon of honey, and sliced almonds.

Mid-morning snack:

Option 1: 1 medium-sized apple and a handful of almonds
Option 2: A hard-boiled Egg with raw carrots and hummus
Option 3: Carrot muffin with a teaspoon of Flaxseeds.

Lunch:

Option 1: Quinoa Salad - Cook 1/2 cup of quinoa with cherry tomatoes, cucumber, and feta cheese with olive oil and lemon juice vinaigrette.
Option 2: Turkey Sandwich - Fill two slices of whole-grain bread with sliced turkey breast, avocado, and veggies. Serve with a small side of roasted sweet potato.
Option 3: Grilled Chicken Salad - Top a salad with grilled chicken breast, cherry tomatoes, feta cheese, and some mixed nuts.

Afternoon snack:

Option 1: 1 cups of Plain Greek yogurt with chopped fruit and mixed nuts

Option 2: A green Smoothie – Blend together a cup of almond milk, 1 banana, 1/2 cup of mixed berries, and a handful of spinach leaves.
Option 3: A Small handful of raisins with raw carrots and hummus.

Dinner:

Option 1: Salmon with quinoa – 5oz of pan-seared Salmon with a side of cooked quinoa, broccoli, and carrots.
Option 2: Beef Taco Bowl with brown rice - Heat 3 oz of beef and top cooked brown rice with shredded lettuce, sliced avocado, and a dollop of salsa.
Option 3: Grilled tofu with vegetables - Marinate tofu and grill alongside mixed vegetables like zucchini, sweet peppers, and tomato.

Snack/Dessert:

Option 1: One serving of Dark chocolate chips with raspberries.

Option 2: A handful of mixed berries with whipped cream.
Option 3: A scoop of frozen yogurt with a serving of granola.

Overall, the fertility diet plan emphasizes a healthy, balanced diet with plenty of fruits and vegetables, lean proteins, whole grains, and healthy fats. It may take some time before you start seeing the benefits of this plan, but with persistence and patience, it may help to improve your reproductive health and increase your chances of conceiving a healthy baby.

Understanding macronutrients and how they contribute to fertility

. Each macronutrient serves a unique purpose in the body, and they all play a significant role in maintaining optimal fertility.

Proteins are critical for fertility because they are the building blocks of all cells in the body, including eggs and sperm. The body breaks down proteins into amino acids, which it uses to repair and regenerate tissues. Proteins are also necessary for the production of hormones, which play a critical role in regulating the menstrual cycle, ovulation, and fertility. Good sources of protein include lean meats, fish, poultry, eggs, legumes, and dairy products.

Carbohydrates are the body's primary source of energy, and they provide fuel for all bodily functions, including reproduction. The body breaks down carbohydrates into glucose, which provides energy to cells. Complex carbohydrates, such as whole grains, fruits, and vegetables, are essential because they release glucose more slowly, providing a steady source of energy. Simple carbohydrates, such as sugar and refined grains, should be avoided as they can cause blood sugar spikes, which can affect fertility.

Fats are essential for various functions in the body, including hormone production, cell growth, and brain function. They also help to regulate inflammation in the body. Omega-3 fatty acids, which are found in fatty fish, nuts, and seeds, are particularly important for fertility because they help to regulate hormones and create a healthy environment for egg and sperm development.

In conclusion, understanding macronutrients and their contributions to fertility is crucial for maintaining optimal reproductive health. A balanced diet that includes plenty of protein, complex carbohydrates, and healthy fats can help to support fertility and improve your chances of conceiving.

Overview of recommended food groups

1. Fruits: Including a variety of fresh, frozen or canned fruits can provide essential vitamins, minerals, and fiber.

2. Vegetables: Eating a variety of vegetables provides nutrients, including potassium, fiber, and vitamins.

3. Grains: Whole grains, such as brown rice, whole wheat bread, and oatmeal, provide fiber, vitamins, and minerals.

4. Protein: Foods like meats, poultry, fish, beans, peas, soy products, and nuts can provide essential nutrients like iron and omega-3 fatty acids.

5. Dairy: Eating low-fat or fat-free dairy products, such as milk, yogurt, and cheese, can provide calcium and other vitamins and minerals.

It is important to eat a variety of foods from each food group to ensure a well-rounded and balanced diet.

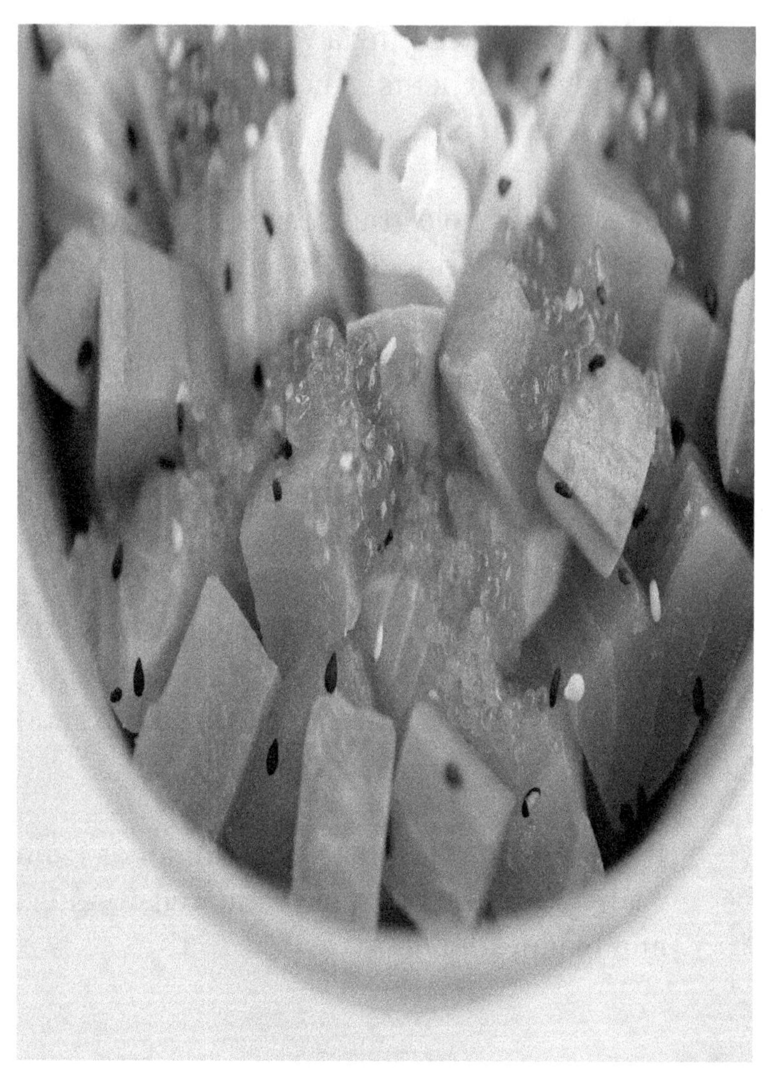

Chapter 3

Recipes for a Healthy Fertility Diet

1. Berry and Yogurt Smoothie: Combine fresh berries, Greek yogurt, and almond milk in a blender for a delicious and nutritious smoothie. Berries are rich in antioxidants, while Greek yogurt is packed with calcium and protein, making this a great breakfast option for fertility health.

2. Avocado and Egg Salad: Combine boiled eggs, mashed avocado, chopped celery, and a dash of lemon juice for a delicious lunch or snack. Avocados are packed with healthy fats and vitamins, while eggs provide a good source of protein.

3. Quinoa Salad with Veggies and Feta Cheese: Combine cooked quinoa, chopped vegetables like bell peppers, tomatoes, cucumbers, and feta cheese for a nutritious and flavorful salad. Quinoa is a good source

of protein and fiber, while vegetables provide essential vitamins and minerals.

4. Grilled Salmon and Asparagus: Season salmon filets with lemon, herbs, and olive oil, then grill alongside asparagus for a healthy and satisfying dinner. Salmon is a good source of omega-3 fatty acids, while asparagus is high in vitamin K and folate.

5. Sweet Potato and Black Bean Tacos: Combine roasted sweet potato cubes with black beans, chopped onions, and jalapenos for a vegetarian and fertility-friendly taco. Sweet potatoes are a good source of vitamin A and fiber, while black beans provide a good source of protein and iron. Enhance the taste by adding avocado and cilantro on top.

Breakfast recipes that are high in fertility-boosting nutrients

1. Avocado and Egg Toast:

Avocado is rich in healthy fats that have been found to promote fertility in both men and women. Adding an egg to this recipe provides protein and vitamin D, which is important for reproductive health.

2. Greek Yogurt Parfait:
Greek yogurt is high in protein and calcium, which are essential nutrients for reproductive health. Adding berries and nuts to the parfait will provide antioxidants and healthy fats.

3. Spinach and Mushroom Omelet:
Spinach is rich in folic acid, which has been linked to increased fertility in women. Mushrooms are also a good source of vitamin D, which has been shown to boost fertility in both men and women.

4. Berry Smoothie:
Berries are high in antioxidants, which help protect reproductive cells from damage. Adding Greek yogurt and honey to the smoothie will provide protein and energy.

5. Steel Cut Oatmeal with Nuts and Fruit:

Oatmeal is a good source of fiber and can help regulate hormone levels, which are crucial for reproductive health. Adding nuts and fruit to the oatmeal will provide healthy fats, antioxidants, and vitamins.

Snack recipes for maintaining energy levels

Here are seven snack recipes that can help you maintain your energy levels:

1. Banana and almond butter bites: Cut banana slices and spread a dollop of almond butter on top of each one. This combination of protein and potassium helps to give you an energy boost.

2. Hard-boiled eggs: This snack option is packed with protein and healthy fats to keep you satiated throughout the day.

3. Greek yogurt with berries: Greek yogurt is an excellent source of protein, and

adding berries will give you an extra burst of energy thanks to the natural sugars.

4. Apple slices with peanut butter: Apples contain natural sugars, while peanut butter provides protein and healthy fats. Together, they make for a perfect energy-packed snack.

5. Hummus and veggie sticks: Hummus is a great source of protein and fiber, while veggies like carrots, celery, and bell peppers provide vitamins and minerals to keep you going.

6. Trail mix: A mixture of nuts, dried fruits, and seeds is a great source of protein, healthy fats, and carbohydrates.

7. Roasted chickpeas: Toss canned chickpeas with olive oil, salt, and your favorite spices and roast them in the oven until crispy. Chickpeas are a good source of fiber and protein, making them a satisfying and energy-boosting snack.

Lunch and dinner recipes that are easy to prepare and nutrient-dense

1. Grilled Salmon with Quinoa Salad: Grill a seasoned salmon filet and serve it with quinoa mixed with chopped tomatoes, cucumbers, and avocado for a flavorful and nutrient-dense meal.

2. Chicken and Sweet Potato Bowls: Roast diced sweet potatoes and grilled chicken breasts and serve them over a bed of spinach with a drizzle of low-fat dressing.

3. Lentil Soup: Cook lentils with vegetables and spices in a slow cooker or on the stove top for an easy soup that's packed with protein and fiber.

4. Black Bean Burrito Bowls: Mix black beans, brown rice, diced tomatoes, and avocado for a filling lunch or dinner.

5. Roasted Vegetables with Brown Rice and Grilled Chicken: Roast veggies like broccoli, bell peppers, and onions and serve them

over brown rice with a grilled chicken breast for a satisfying and nutrient-rich meal.

6. Quinoa and Kale Salad: Mix cooked quinoa with chopped kale, avocado, and roasted walnuts for a salad that's high in protein, healthy fats, and fiber.

7. Baked Sweet Potato Fries with Turkey Burgers: Make sweet potato fries by slicing sweet potatoes into wedges and baking them in the oven. Serve them with grilled turkey burgers for a healthy and satisfying dinner.

8. Vegetarian Chili: Make a big pot of chili with beans, vegetables, and spices and serve it with a side of whole-grain bread for a hearty and nutritious meal.

Recipes for healthy desserts to satisfy sweet cravings

1. Chocolate avocado pudding - Blend together one ripe avocado, ¼ cup of cacao powder, ¼ cup of almond milk and sweetener of your choice (honey, maple syrup or stevia) until smooth. Chill for an hour before serving.

2. Berry and yogurt parfait - In a cup, layer a combination of Greek yogurt, fresh berries (strawberries, blueberries, and raspberries), honey and granola. Repeat layers and top with additional fruit.

3. Banana oat cookies – Mash two ripe bananas and mix in 1 cup of rolled oats and 2 tablespoons of honey. Bake at 350 degrees Fahrenheit until golden brown (around 15-20 minutes).

4. Chocolate chip energy bites - Combine 1 cup of rolled oats, ½ cup of peanut butter, 1/3 cup of honey, ½ teaspoon of vanilla

extract, and ¼ cup of mini chocolate chips in a bowl. Roll mixture into bite-size balls and store in the refrigerator.

5. Baked apples – Slice a whole apple into small pieces, and sprinkle with cinnamon and honey. Bake in the oven for 15-20 minutes and serve with a dollop of Greek yogurt or whipped cream.

6. Chia seed pudding – Mix 1/3 cup of chia seeds with 1 cup of coconut milk and 1 tablespoon of honey. Let sit in the refrigerator overnight, then top with fresh fruit and granola.

7. Banana almond butter cups - Mix 1 ripe banana and 1/3 cup of almond butter together. Pour the mixture into a mini muffin pan and freeze. Once set, remove from the pan and drizzle with melted dark chocolate.

8. Frozen yogurt bark - Mix 2 cups of Greek yogurt, 1 tablespoon of honey and 1 cup of chopped fruit. Spread the mixture onto a baking sheet lined with parchment paper and freeze. After it solidifies, divide it into fragments and relish it.

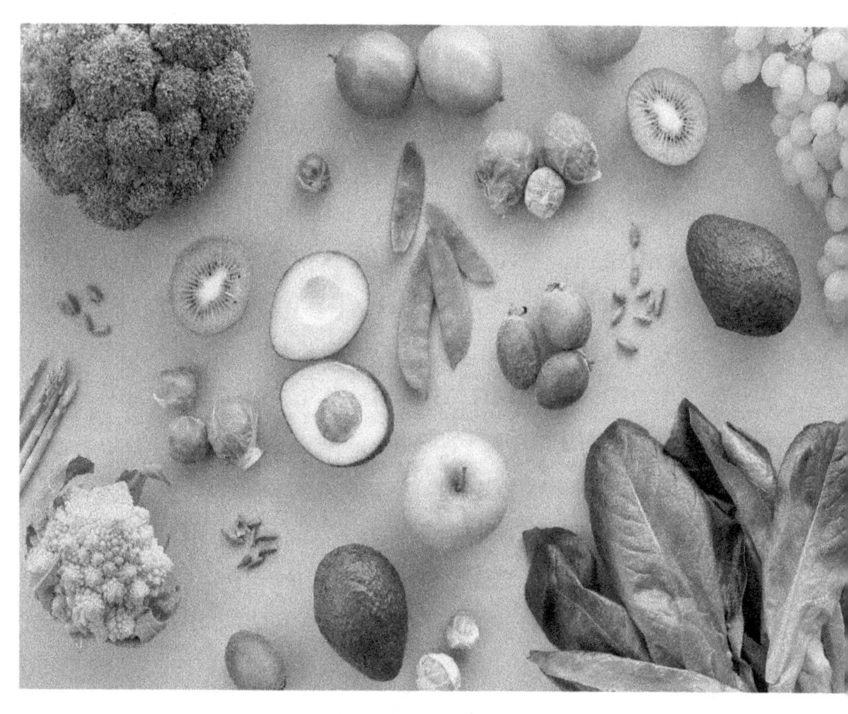

Chapter 4

Additional Strategies for Fertility

1. Maintain a healthy body weight: Being overweight or underweight can affect fertility. A healthy body weight can positively impact fertility by promoting hormonal balance and optimizing ovulation.

2. Stop smoking and limit alcohol intake: Both smoking and excessive alcohol intake have negative effects on fertility in both men and women.

3. Get enough sleep: Sleep deprivation can affect hormonal balance, which can affect fertility. It is essential to get enough sleep to reduce stress levels.

4. Reduce stress: High levels of stress can reduce fertility in both men and women. Finding ways to manage stress, such as

practicing relaxation techniques, exercising, and taking breaks, can help.

5. Consider dietary changes: A balanced diet can positively impact fertility. Foods rich in antioxidants, omega-3 fatty acids, and folic acid can improve overall fertility.

6. Manage pre-existing conditions: Pre-existing medical conditions like PCOS, thyroid disorders, and diabetes can affect fertility. Consulting a doctor can help manage these conditions.

7. Regular exercise: Exercise can help maintain a healthy body weight, reduce stress and improve overall health, which can positively affect fertility.

8. Seek medical help: If you have been trying to conceive without success, consulting a fertility specialist may help identify any underlying issues or recommend fertility treatments to achieve pregnancy.

The importance of exercise and stress management for fertility

Both exercise and stress management are critical factors that can affect fertility in various ways. Exercise helps promote fertility by improving blood circulation, increasing oxygen supply to the reproductive organs, reducing inflammation, and balancing insulin levels. Regular exercise also helps in maintaining a healthy weight, which is crucial for fertility in both women and men.

Stress, on the other hand, can impact fertility negatively by altering the hormonal balance, causing irregular menstrual cycles, lowering libido, and lowering the chances of conception. Stress management techniques such as meditation, deep breathing exercises, or yoga can help reduce stress and improve overall well-being.

In conclusion, exercise and stress management are essential factors in promoting fertility. Couples seeking to conceive should aim to maintain a healthy and active lifestyle while incorporating stress-reducing efforts into their daily routines.

Tips for creating a healthy lifestyle conducive to fertility

1. Maintain a healthy weight: Being overweight or underweight can interfere with hormone production and lead to irregular periods, making it harder to conceive. To sustain a healthy weight, it is recommended to follow a well-balanced diet and engage in regular exercise.

2. Quit smoking: Smoking can damage fertility in both men and women. Ceasing smoking may enhance fertility and augment the possibility of succeeding in conceiving a child.

3. Cut down on alcohol: Alcohol can affect fertility in both men and women. It's advised to cut down on alcohol

consumption or avoid it altogether if you're trying to conceive.

4. Manage stress: High levels of stress can cause hormonal imbalances that can interfere with ovulation. Incorporate stress management methods such as meditation, yoga, or deep breathing exercises into your daily routine.

5. Get enough sleep: Lack of sleep can affect the reproductive system and interfere with hormonal balance. Strive to acquire a minimum of seven hours of sleep every night.

6. Avoid exposure to toxins: Exposure to chemicals and toxins can harm fertility. Avoid harmful chemicals and toxins in your environment and be cautious with the use of products containing BPA, such as plastic bottles.

7. Take prenatal vitamins: Taking prenatal vitamins with folic acid can support healthy fetal development and increase the chances of conception.

8. Stay hydrated: Staying hydrated is important for reproductive health. Consume ample amounts of water and restrict the consumption of sugary beverages.

9. Visit your doctor regularly: Regular check-ups with your doctor can help identify any potential fertility issues and address them early on.

10. Be patient: Conceiving can take time, and stress and anxiety can make it harder. Remember to stay positive and patient throughout the process and seek support from loved ones if needed.

Fertility supplements and their roles on reproductive health

Fertility supplements are dietary supplements that aim to improve reproductive health and increase the chances of conception. These supplements contain a variety of vitamins, minerals, herbs, and other natural ingredients that are believed to support fertility by addressing nutrient deficiencies, hormonal imbalances, and other factors that can affect reproductive function. Some of the most common fertility supplements and their roles in reproductive health are:

1. Folic acid: Folic acid is a type of B vitamin that is essential for the development of a healthy fetus. It helps to prevent neural tube defects and other birth defects that can occur in the early stages of pregnancy. Folic acid also supports ovulation and aids in the production of healthy eggs.

2. Omega-3 fatty acids: Omega-3 fatty acids are essential fatty acids that play a vital role in reproductive health. They help to regulate hormones, reduce inflammation, and improve egg quality. Omega-3 fatty acids can be found in fish oil supplements and certain types of food, such as salmon and flaxseed.

3. Coenzyme Q10: Coenzyme Q10 is an antioxidant that is essential for energy production in cells. It is also believed to improve male fertility by boosting sperm quality and motility.

4. Vitamin D: Vitamin D plays a crucial role in the development and health of the reproductive system. It helps to regulate hormone production and improve egg quality. Vitamin D deficiency has been linked to infertility and pregnancy complications.

5. Maca Root: Maca root is a Peruvian herb that has been used for centuries as a fertility aid. It is believed to improve libido, regulate hormones, and increase sperm count.

Overall, fertility supplements can play an important role in supporting reproductive health and increasing the chances of conception. It is crucial to consult with a healthcare professional prior to taking any supplements, as they may have adverse reactions with medication and cause potential side effects.

Conclusion

Based on the research on the "fertility diet," it can be concluded that following a healthy and balanced diet can improve a woman's chances of conception. The fertility diet plan outlined in the cookbook emphasizes consuming more whole foods, vegetables, fruits, and whole grains and limiting processed foods, caffeine, and alcohol. Additionally, the cookbook provides recipes that support the recommended nutrient intake for women trying to conceive.

Overall, the fertility diet cookbook plan is a well-designed program that promotes healthy eating habits, which can benefit women's reproductive health. However, it is essential to recognize that the cookbook should not replace medical advice from a fertility specialist or doctor. Women should also consider other factors that may impact their fertility, such as genetics, age, and overall health. In conclusion, incorporating the fertility diet in conjunction with medical advice, exercise, and stress management can potentially improve a woman's chance of conceiving.

- Recap of the importance of nutrition for fertility

Nutrition plays a crucial role in fertility by impacting both male and female reproductive functions. A balanced and nutritious diet is essential for improving fertility outcomes, as it can enhance hormonal balance, improve egg and sperm quality, promote regular menstrual cycles, and reduce the risk of infertility problems. Proper nutrition can also decrease the likelihood of developing chronic diseases that can lead to fertility problems. Understanding the impact of nutrition on fertility can provide individuals and couples with the knowledge they need to make informed choices about their diet and optimize their chances of conceiving.

Final thoughts and advice for women trying to conceive

1. Be patient and keep an open mind: It's important to remember that conception can take time, and that it's possible for it to happen naturally without any interventions.

2. Maintain a healthy lifestyle: Follow a balanced and nutritious diet, engage in regular exercise, manage stress levels, avoid smoking and excessive alcohol and caffeine consumption.

3. Stay informed and seek help: Learn about fertility and the factors that can affect it, keep track of your menstrual cycles, and seek medical advice if you have concerns or if you've been trying to conceive for a year without success.

4. Surround yourself with support: Lean on your partner, friends, and family, or join a support group for women trying to conceive.

5. Be positive and hopeful: Believe in your body's ability to conceive and try to maintain a positive outlook through the ups and downs of the journey to becoming a parent.